PARKINSON'S DIET COOKBOOK

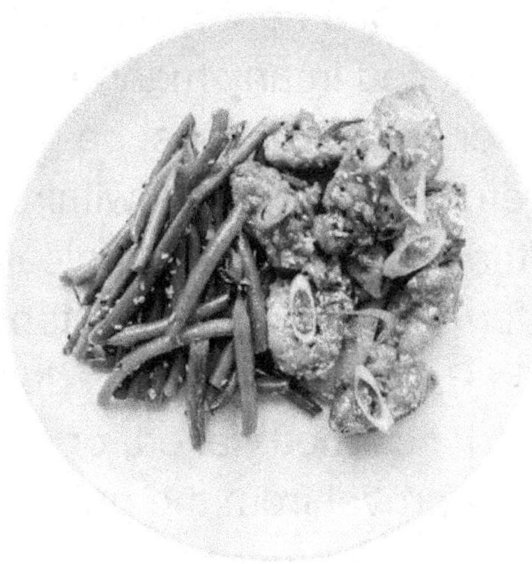

Recipes for Healthy Living and Management of Neurological Diseases

Anita Mark

DISCLAIMER

Copyright © by (Anita Mark 2024). All rights reserved.

Acknowledgment

I extend my heartfelt appreciation to all those who have contributed to the creation of this cookbook, "Parkinson's Diet Cookbook."

To the individuals living with Parkinson's disease, whose courage and resilience have inspired every page of this book, thank you for sharing your stories and experiences.

To the caregivers, families, and loved ones who provide unwavering support and care for those affected by Parkinson's, your dedication is truly commendable.

To the healthcare professionals and researchers who tirelessly work to improve the lives of individuals with Parkinson's, your expertise and guidance have been invaluable.

To my family and friends, thank you for your encouragement and understanding throughout this journey.

And to the readers, may the recipes and insights within this cookbook bring comfort, nourishment, and hope to your lives.

With gratitude,

[Anita Mark]

DEDICATION

This cookbook is dedicated to all those touched by Parkinson's disease may it serve as a beacon of hope and empowerment on your journey to wellness. To the individuals living with Parkinson's, their caregivers, and their loved ones, this book is a testament to your strength, resilience, and unwavering spirit. And to the healthcare professionals, researchers, and advocates who tirelessly work to improve the lives of those affected by Parkinson's, your dedication is truly commendable. With heartfelt appreciation and unwavering dedication, this book is lovingly dedicated to you.

[Anita Mark]

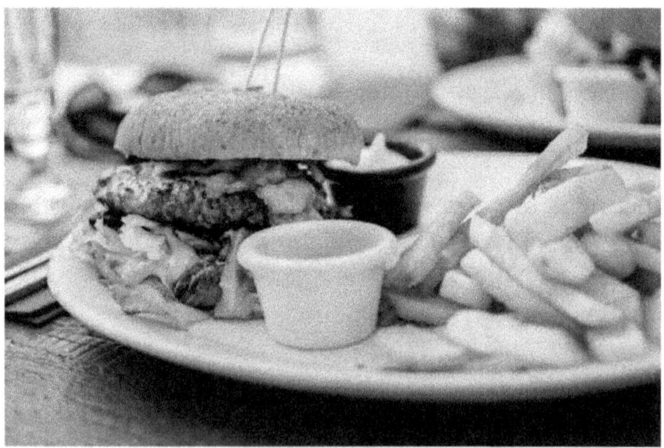

Table of Contents

Introduction

As I sat in the doctor's office, my hands trembled involuntarily. The neurologist's words echoed in my mind, "You have Parkinson's disease." Shock coursed through me like an electric current, leaving me numb and overwhelmed.

My journey with Parkinson's began with subtle signs that I initially brushed off as mere quirks of aging. A slight tremor in my hand, stiffness in my limbs, and a 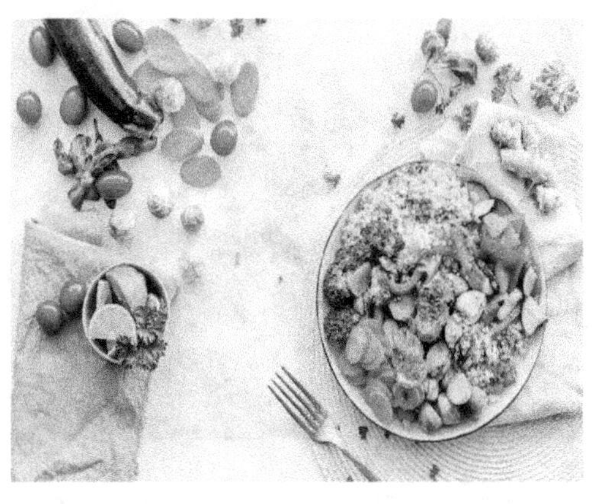 gradual loss of balance. I attributed these symptoms to stress or fatigue, never suspecting the underlying cause.

However, as time passed, the symptoms intensified, interfering with my daily activities and eroding my quality of life. Simple tasks like buttoning a shirt or pouring a glass of water became daunting challenges.

Concerned, I sought medical advice, hoping for reassurance and a quick fix.

The diagnosis shattered my world. Parkinson's disease is a progressive neurological disorder with no cure. The news hit me like a sledgehammer, leaving me grappling with a whirlwind of emotions – fear, anger, and despair. Questions flooded my mind relentlessly. How would this impact my career, my relationships, my future?

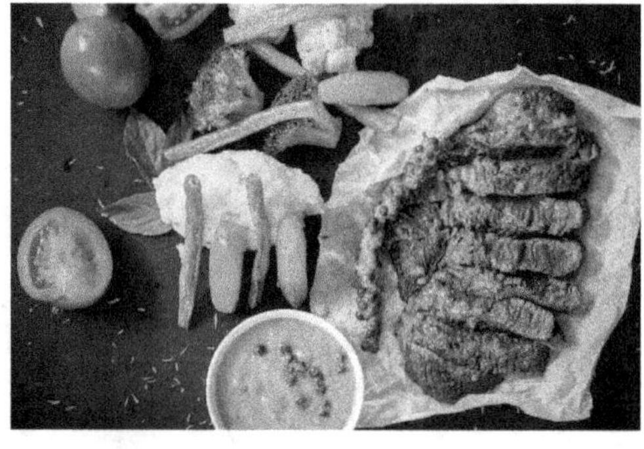

Navigating the aftermath of diagnosis was akin to treading uncharted waters. I oscillated between denial and acceptance, wrestling with the harsh reality of my new reality. Each day brought its own set of challenges, from adjusting to medication regimens to coping with fluctuating symptoms.

Despite the overwhelming uncertainty, I refused to succumb to despair. Armed with resilience and determination, I embarked on a journey of adaptation. I sought solace in the Parkinson's community, finding camaraderie and support among fellow warriors battling the same foe.

Embracing an active lifestyle became my cornerstone in the fight against Parkinson's. I prioritized regular exercise, incorporating activities like walking, yoga, and tai chi into my daily routine. Physical therapy sessions helped alleviate stiffness and improve mobility, empowering me to reclaim control over my body.

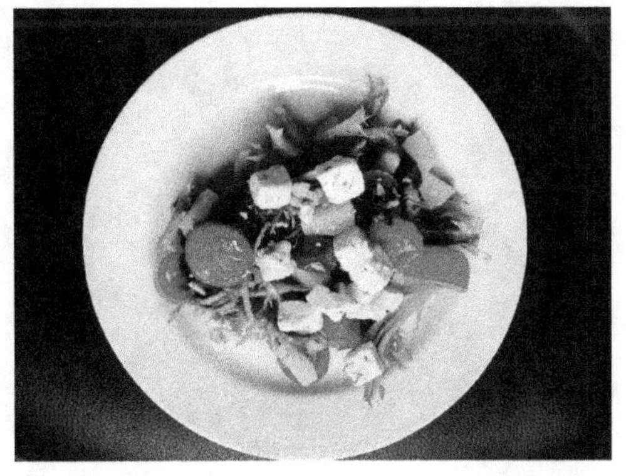

Equally pivotal was adopting a balanced diet tailored to my specific needs as a Parkinson's patient. Nutrient-rich foods became my allies in combating symptoms and promoting overall well-being. I discovered the profound impact of diet on my energy levels, cognition, and mood, fueling my determination to make healthy choices a priority.

Though Parkinson's imposed its share of obstacles, it also served as a catalyst for personal growth and resilience. I learned to cherish life's simple joys, finding beauty in moments of stillness and gratitude. Each day presents its own set of challenges, but I face them with unwavering resolve and an indomitable spirit. Parkinson's may have changed the course of my journey, but it will never define who I am or what I am capable of achieving.

Understanding Parkinson's Disease

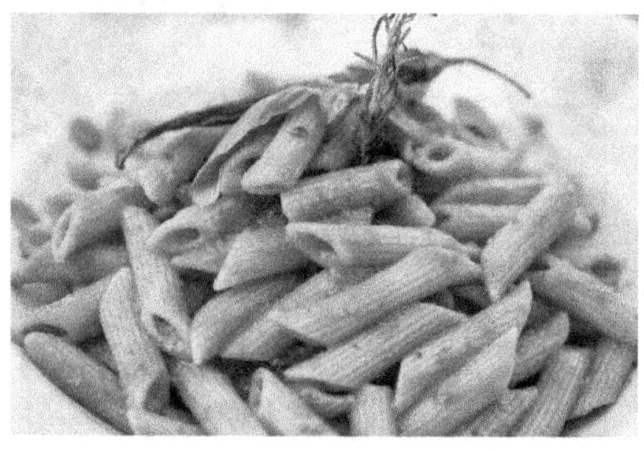

Parkinson's disease is a progressive neurological disorder that affects movement. It occurs when nerve cells in the brain that produce dopamine, a chemical messenger responsible for coordinating muscle movement, become damaged or die. As dopamine levels decrease, individuals experience a range of motor symptoms, including tremors, stiffness, slowness of movement, and impaired balance and coordination. In addition to motor symptoms, Parkinson's can also cause nonmotor symptoms such as cognitive changes, mood disturbances, sleep disturbances, and autonomic dysfunction. While the exact cause of Parkinson's disease is unknown, factors such as genetics, environmental toxins, and oxidative stress are believed to play a role. Currently, there is no cure for Parkinson's, but treatments such as medication, surgery, and lifestyle modifications can help manage symptoms and improve the quality of life for individuals living with the condition. Early diagnosis and comprehensive care are crucial in effectively managing the progression of the disease.

Symptoms of Parkinson's Disease

1.   Tremors: Involuntary shaking, usually starting in one hand, which may occur while the individual's body is at rest. Tremors are often one of the 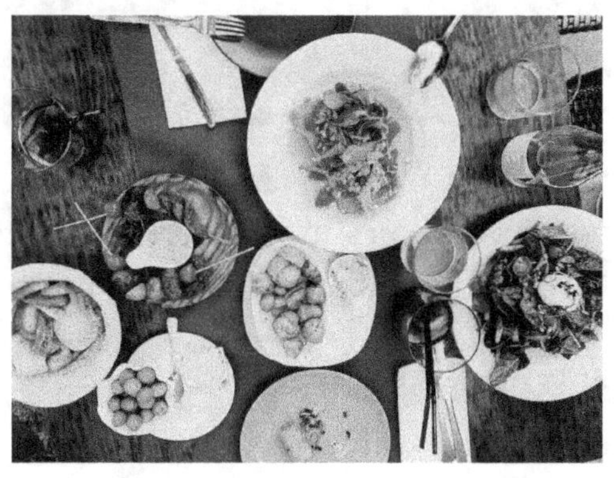 first symptoms noticed in Parkinson's.

2. Bradykinesia: Slowness of movement, making simple tasks such as buttoning a shirt or walking difficult and time-consuming. It can also affect facial expressions, resulting in a lack of spontaneous movement (hypomimia).

3. Rigidity: Stiffness and inflexibility of muscles, which can lead to decreased range of motion and joint pain. Rigidity often affects the limbs but can also occur in the neck and trunk muscles.

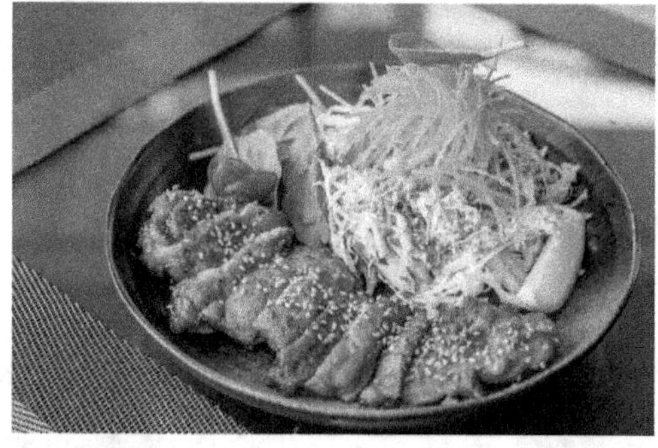

4. Postural instability: Impaired balance and coordination, leading to difficulty in maintaining an upright posture and an increased risk of falls. Individuals with Parkinson's may experience a stooped posture and have trouble with gait (walking pattern).

5. Bradyphrenia: Cognitive changes, including difficulties with memory, concentration, and executive function. Parkinson's can affect cognitive abilities such as planning, problem-solving, and multitasking.

6. Freezing: Brief episodes where a person feels stuck in place and unable to initiate movement, particularly when starting to walk or turning around.

7. Micrographia: Small, cramped handwriting that becomes increasingly difficult to read as the disease progresses.

8. Speech changes: Soft, monotone voice (hypophonia) and slurred or hesitant speech

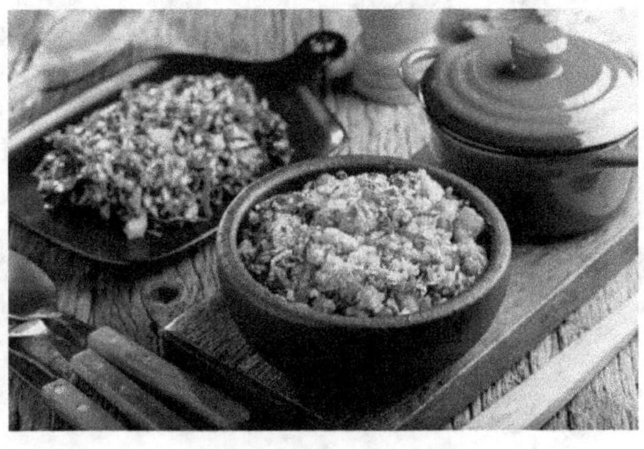

(dysarthria) are common in Parkinson's disease due to changes in the muscles involved in speech production.

9. Nonmotor symptoms: Parkinson's can also cause a range of nonmotor symptoms, including depression, anxiety, sleep disturbances, constipation, urinary problems, and changes in the sense of smell.

It's important to note that Parkinson's symptoms can vary widely among individuals, and not everyone will experience all of these symptoms. Additionally, the severity and progression of symptoms can differ from person to person. Early diagnosis and personalized treatment plans can help manage symptoms and improve the quality of life for individuals living with Parkinson's disease.

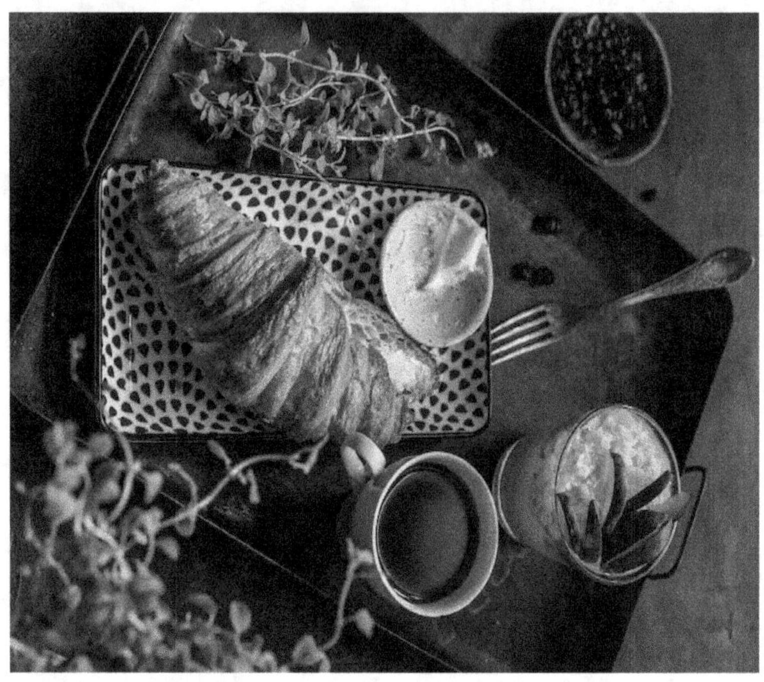

Nutritional Guidelines for Parkinson's Patients

Key nutritional guidelines for Parkinson's patients include:

1. Balanced Diet: Aim for a well-balanced diet rich in fruits, vegetables, whole grains, lean proteins, and healthy fats. This provides essential nutrients for overall health and supports optimal brain function.

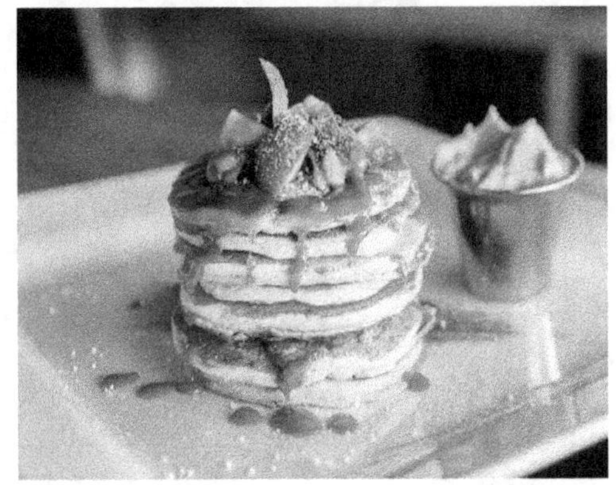

2. Protein Distribution: Distribute protein intake evenly throughout the day, rather than consuming large amounts in one meal. This can help minimize the impact of protein on the absorption of Parkinson's medications, which contain levodopa.

3. Adequate Hydration: Drink plenty of fluids throughout the day to stay hydrated. Dehydration can worsen symptoms such as constipation and urinary problems, which are common in Parkinson's.

4. FiberRich Foods: Include fiber-rich foods such as fruits, vegetables, whole grains, and legumes in your diet to promote digestive health and prevent constipation, a common symptom of Parkinson's disease.

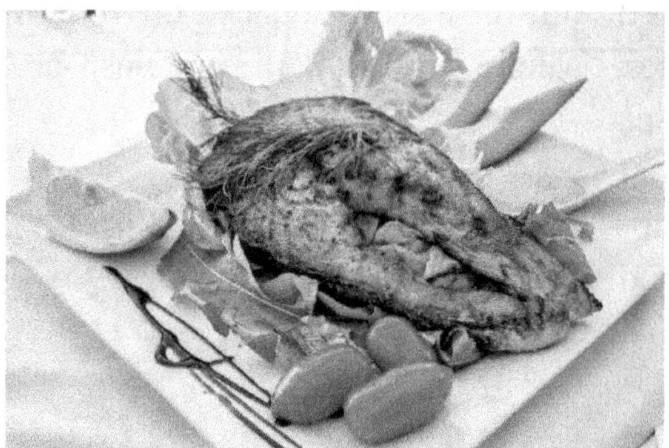

5. Limit Saturated and Trans Fats: Limit intake of saturated and trans fats found in fried foods, processed snacks, and fatty meats. Instead, choose healthier fats such as those found in nuts, seeds, avocados, and olive oil.

6. Monitor Medication Timing: Be mindful of the timing of medication and meals. Some Parkinson's medications should be taken on an empty stomach for optimal absorption, while others may be taken with food to reduce side effects such as nausea.

7. Vitamin D and Calcium: Ensure adequate intake of vitamin D and calcium to support bone health. Vitamin D can be obtained from sunlight exposure and fortified foods, while calcium-rich foods include dairy products, leafy greens, and fortified plant-based alternatives.

8. Consider Supplements: Consult with a healthcare professional or registered dietitian to determine if supplements such as vitamin B12, omega-3 fatty acids, or antioxidants

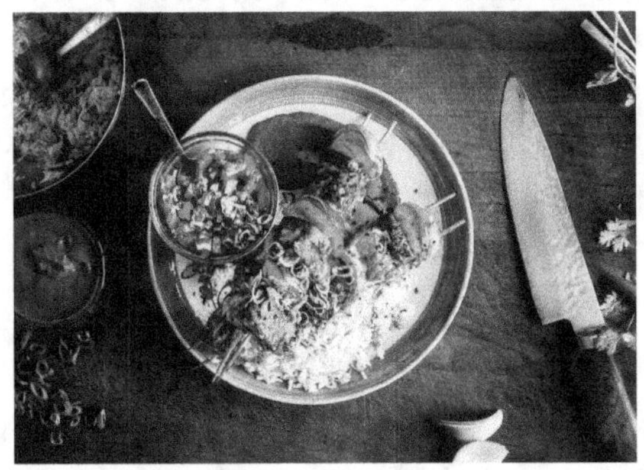

are appropriate for your individual needs.

9. Be Mindful of Swallowing Difficulties: If swallowing difficulties (dysphagia) are present, modify food texture and consistency as needed to reduce the risk of choking or aspiration. Soft, moist foods and thickened liquids may be easier to swallow.

10. Monitor Weight: Keep track of your weight and consult with a healthcare professional if you experience unintended weight loss or gain. Maintaining a healthy weight is important for overall health and can help manage symptoms of Parkinson's disease.

By following these nutritional guidelines, individuals with Parkinson's disease can support their overall health and well-being while managing symptoms and optimizing medication effectiveness. It's essential to work with healthcare professionals, including a neurologist and registered dietitian, to develop a personalized nutrition plan tailored to individual needs and preferences.

Foods to Include and foods to avoid as Parkinson's patients

Foods to Include:

1. Fruits and Vegetables: Rich in vitamins, minerals, and antioxidants, fruits and vegetables support overall health and may help reduce inflammation. To guarantee a wide spectrum of nutrients, aim for a range of colors.

2. Whole Grains: Choose whole grains such as brown rice, quinoa, oats, and whole wheat bread and pasta. These provide fiber for digestive health and sustained energy release.

3. Lean Proteins: Opt for lean protein sources such as skinless poultry, fish, tofu, beans, lentils, and eggs. For the health and regeneration of muscles, protein is necessary.

4. Healthy Fats: Include sources of healthy fats, such as nuts, seeds, avocados, and olive oil. These fats support brain health and may help reduce inflammation.

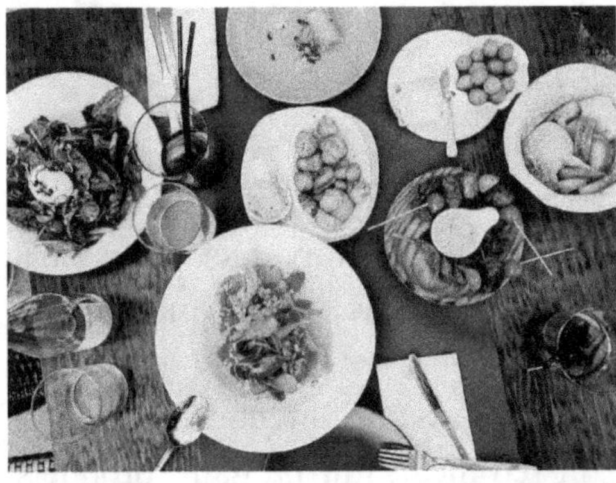

5. Omega3 Fatty Acids: Incorporate omega-3 rich foods such as fatty fish (salmon, mackerel, sardines), flaxseeds, chia seeds, and walnuts. Omega3 fatty acids have anti-inflammatory properties and may benefit brain function.

6. Water: Stay hydrated by drinking plenty of water throughout the day. Proper hydration supports digestion, cognitive function, and overall well-being.

7. CalciumRich Foods: Ensure adequate intake of calcium through dairy products, fortified plant-based alternatives, leafy greens, and nuts. Calcium is important for bone health, especially for individuals at risk of osteoporosis.

8. Vitamin D Sources: Get vitamin D from sunlight exposure, fortified foods (such as fortified milk and cereals), and supplements if necessary. Vitamin D supports bone health and may have neuroprotective effects.

Foods to Avoid or Limit:

1. Processed Foods: Minimize intake of processed foods high in sodium, sugar, and unhealthy fats. These can contribute to inflammation and exacerbate symptoms.

2. Saturated and Trans Fats: Limit consumption of saturated fats found in red meat, full-fat dairy products, and fried foods, as well as trans fats found in processed snacks and baked goods. These fats can increase inflammation and cardiovascular risk.

3. Excessive Protein: While protein is important, consuming large amounts in one meal may interfere with the absorption of Parkinson's medications containing levodopa. Make sure your daily protein intake is spread equally.

4. Caffeine and Alcohol: Limit intake of caffeine and alcohol, as they can affect sleep quality, exacerbate tremors, and interact with Parkinson's medications.

5. Heavy Meals: Avoid heavy, large meals, especially in the evening, as they may worsen digestion and interfere with sleep. Rather, choose to eat smaller, more often.

By focusing on a balanced diet rich in nutrient-dense foods and minimizing intake of processed and unhealthy options, individuals with Parkinson's disease can support their overall health and well-being while managing symptoms effectively. It's important to consult with a healthcare professional or registered dietitian for personalized dietary recommendations based on individual needs and preferences.

Chapter One: Parkinson's Diet Appetizers

Stuffed Mushrooms

Ingredients:

12 large mushrooms (such as cremini or button)
8 oz cream cheese, softened
1/4 cup chopped spinach
2 cloves garlic, minced
1/4 cup grated Parmesan cheese

Preparation Time: 15 minutes
Cooking Time: 1520 minutes
Method of Preparation:

1. Preheat the oven to 350°F (175°C).
2. Cut the mushrooms into tiny pieces after removing the stems.
3. In a mixing bowl, combine cream cheese, chopped spinach, minced garlic, chopped mushroom stems, and grated Parmesan cheese.
4. Insert the cream cheese mixture into the caps of each mushroom.

5. Place stuffed mushrooms on a baking sheet and bake for 15-20 minutes, or until mushrooms are tender and the filling is bubbly.

Nutrition Information (per serving):
Calories: 80
Protein: 4g
Carbohydrates: 2g
Fat: 6g

Serving Size: 3 stuffed mushrooms per person

Caprese Skewers:

Ingredients:

Cherry tomatoes
Fresh mozzarella balls
Basil leaves
Balsamic glaze (optional)

Preparation Time: 10 minutes
Method of Preparation:

1. Attach a basil leaf, a mozzarella ball, and a cherry tomato to little skewers.
2. Arrange the skewers on a plate and drizzle with balsamic glaze, if desired.

Nutrition Information (per serving):

Calories: 120
Protein: 6g
Carbohydrates: 3g
Fat: 8g

Serving Size: 3 skewers per person

Smoked Salmon RollUps:

Ingredients:

Smoked salmon slices
Cream cheese
Cucumber strips
Fresh dill (optional)

Preparation Time: 10 minutes
Method of Preparation:

1. Spread a thin layer of cream cheese on each smoked salmon slice.

2. Place a cucumber strip on one end of the salmon slice and roll up tightly.

3. Secure with a toothpick and garnish with fresh dill, if desired.

Nutrition Information (per serving):

Calories: 90
Protein: 5g
Carbohydrates: 2g
Fat: 7g

Serving Size: 2 rollups per person

<u>Cucumber Avocado Rolls:</u>

Ingredients:

Cucumber
Avocado
Smoked salmon or cooked shrimp (optional)
Thinly sliced radish (optional)

Preparation Time: 15 minutes
Method of Preparation:

1. Using a vegetable peeler, slice the cucumber lengthwise into thin strips.
2. Spread mashed avocado onto each cucumber strip.
3. Top with smoked salmon or cooked shrimp and thinly sliced radish, if desired.
4. Roll up the cucumber strips and secure with a toothpick.

Nutrition Information (per serving):

Calories: 110
Protein: 3g
Carbohydrates: 6g
Fat: 8g

Serving Size: 4 rolls per persons

<u>Deviled Eggs:</u>

Ingredients:

Hard Boiled eggs
Mayonnaise or Greek yogurt
Dijon mustard
Paprika
Chopped chives (optional)

Preparation Time: 15 minutes

Method of Preparation:

1. Slice hard-boiled eggs in half lengthwise and remove the yolks.

2. Mash the yolks with mayonnaise or Greek yogurt, Dijon mustard, and a pinch of paprika until smooth.

3. Spoon or pipe the yolk mixture back into the egg white halves.

4. Garnish with chopped chives and additional paprika, if desired.

Nutrition Information (per serving):

Calories: 70
Protein: 6g
Carbohydrates: 1g

Fat: 5g

Serving Size: 2 halves per person

These appetizer recipes are delicious, nutritious, and easy to prepare, making them perfect for individuals with Parkinson's disease. Enjoy them as starters for meals or as snacks for gatherings and events. Changes can be made in accordance with dietary requirements and personal preferences.

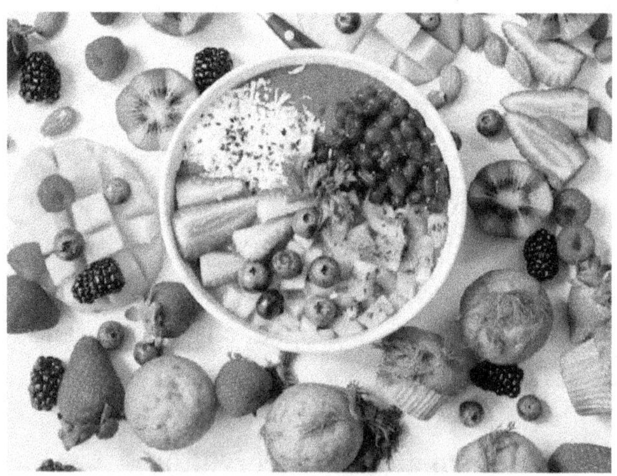

Chapter Two: Parkinson's Diet Soups

Creamy Tomato Basil Soup:

Ingredients:

1 tablespoon olive oil
1 onion, chopped
2 cloves garlic, minced
Two cans of diced tomatoes, 14.5 ounces each
1 tablespoon tomato paste
2 cups low-sodium vegetable broth
1/2 cup fresh basil leaves, chopped
1/2 cup plain Greek yogurt (or coconut cream for dairy free option)
Salt and pepper to taste

Preparation Time: 10 minutes
Cooking Time: 25 minutes

Method of Preparation:

1. Place a big saucepan over medium heat with olive oil. Add chopped onion and minced garlic, and sauté until softened about 5 minutes.

2. Add diced tomatoes (with their juices) and tomato paste to the pot. Stir to combine.

3. Pour in vegetable broth and bring the mixture to a simmer. Give it a good 15 to 20 minutes to cook so the flavors can combine.

4. Remove the pot from heat and use an immersion blender to puree the soup until smooth.

5. Stir in chopped basil leaves and Greek yogurt (or coconut cream). Season with salt and pepper to taste.

6. Return the pot to low heat and simmer for an additional 5 minutes.

7. Serve hot, garnished with additional basil leaves if desired.

Nutrition Information (per serving):

Calories: 120
Protein: 4g
Carbohydrates: 14g
Fat: 6g
Fiber: 3g
Sugar: 8g
Sodium: 400mg
Serving Size: 1 cup

<u>Chicken and Vegetable Soup:</u>

Ingredients:

1 tablespoon olive oil
1 onion, chopped
2 carrots, diced
2 celery stalks, diced
2 cloves garlic, minced
4 cups low-sodium chicken broth
Two cups of shredded cooked chicken breast
1 cup frozen peas
Salt and pepper to taste
Fresh parsley for garnish

Preparation Time: 15 minutes
Cooking Time: 25 minutes

Method of Preparation:

1. Place a big saucepan over medium heat and add the olive oil. Incorporate diced celery, diced carrots, diced onion, and minced garlic. Cook for 5 to 7 minutes, or until veggies are tender.

2. Pour in chicken broth and bring the mixture to a simmer. Give it a good 15 to 20 minutes to cook so the flavors can combine.

3. Add shredded chicken breast and frozen peas to the pot. Cook for an additional 5 minutes, until chicken is heated through and peas are tender.

4. To taste, add salt and pepper for seasoning.

5. If preferred, top the dish with fresh parsley.

Nutrition Information (per serving):

Calories: 180
Protein: 20g
Carbohydrates: 10g
Fat: 6g
Fiber: 3g
Sugar: 4g
Sodium: 500mg

Serving Size: 1 cup

<u>Vegetable Lentil Soup:</u>

Ingredients:

1 tablespoon olive oil
1 onion, chopped
2 carrots, diced
2 celery stalks, diced
2 cloves garlic, minced
1 cup dried green lentils, rinsed
4 cups low-sodium vegetable broth
A single 14.5 oz can of chopped tomatoes
1 teaspoon dried thyme
1 teaspoon dried oregano
Salt and pepper to taste
Fresh parsley for garnish

Preparation Time: 15 minutes
Cooking Time: 30 minutes

Method of Preparation:

1. Place a big saucepan over medium heat with olive oil. Add the minced garlic, diced celery, diced carrots, and sliced onion. Sauté the vegetables for 5 to 7 minutes, or until they are tender.

2. Add dried lentils, vegetable broth, diced tomatoes (with their juices), dried thyme, and dried oregano to the pot. Stir to combine.

3. Bring the mixture to a boil, then reduce heat to low. Lentils should be soft after 20 to 25 minutes of simmering under cover.

4. Add pepper and salt to taste.

5. If preferred, top the dish with fresh parsley.

Nutrition Information (per serving):

Calories: 200

Protein: 12g

Carbohydrates: 32g

Fat: 3g

Fiber: 12g

Sugar: 6g

Sodium: 600mg

Serving Size: 1 cup

<u>Butternut Squash Soup</u>

Ingredients:

1 tablespoon olive oil
1 onion, chopped
One chopped, peeled, and seeded butternut squash
2 carrots, diced
2 cloves garlic, minced
4 cups low-sodium vegetable broth
1 teaspoon ground cumin
1/2 teaspoon ground cinnamon
Salt and pepper to taste
Pumpkin seeds for garnish (optional)

Preparation Time: 20 minutes
Cooking Time: 25 minutes
Method of Preparation:

1. Place a big saucepan over medium heat with olive oil. Add chopped onion and minced garlic. Sauté until softened, about 5 minutes.

2. Add diced butternut squash, diced carrots, vegetable broth, ground cumin, and ground cinnamon to the pot. Stir to combine.

3. Bring the mixture to a boil, then reduce heat to low. Cover and simmer for 20-25 minutes, or until vegetables are tender.

4. Puree the soup with an immersion blender until it's completely creamy. Alternatively, transfer the soup to a blender and blend in batches until smooth.

5. Season with salt and pepper to taste.

6. Serve hot, garnished with pumpkin seeds if desired.

Nutrition Information (per serving):

Calories: 150
Protein: 3g
Carbohydrates: 30g
Fat: 4g
Fiber: 6g
Sugar: 6g
Sodium: 500mg

Serving Size: 1 cup

Of course! Here are two additional Parkinson's Friendly soup recipes:

Spinach and White Bean Soup:

Ingredients:

1 tablespoon olive oil
1 onion, chopped
2 cloves garlic, minced
4 cups low-sodium vegetable broth
Two cans of rinsed and drained white beans, 15 ounces each
4 cups fresh spinach leaves
1 teaspoon dried thyme
Salt and pepper to taste
Lemon wedges for serving (optional)

Preparation Time: 10 minutes
Cooking Time: 20 minutes

Method of Preparation:

1. Place a big saucepan over medium heat with olive oil. Add chopped onion and minced garlic. Sauté until softened, about 5 minutes.

2. Add vegetable broth, white beans, and dried thyme to the pot. Simmer for ten minutes after bringing to a simmer.

3. Stir in fresh spinach leaves and continue to simmer for another 5 minutes, or until the spinach is wilted.

4. Use an immersion blender to partially blend the soup, leaving some beans whole for texture.

5. Season with salt and pepper to taste.

6. Serve hot, with lemon wedges on the side for squeezing over the soup if desired.

Nutrition Information (per serving):

Calories: 180
Protein: 9g
Carbohydrates: 30g
Fat: 3g
Fiber: 9g
Sugar: 2g
Sodium: 600mg

Serving Size: 1 cup

<u>Mushroom Barley Soup:</u>

Ingredients:

1 tablespoon olive oil
1 onion, chopped
2 cloves garlic, minced
8 oz mushrooms, sliced
1 cup pearl barley, rinsed
6 cups low-sodium vegetable broth
1 teaspoon dried thyme
Salt and pepper to taste
Chopped fresh parsley for garnish

Preparation Time: 15 minutes
Cooking Time: 40 minutes

Method of Preparation:

1. Place a big saucepan over medium heat with olive oil. Add chopped onion and minced garlic. Sauté until softened, about 5 minutes.

2. Add sliced mushrooms to the pot and cook until they release their juices and begin to brown about 7-8 minutes.

3. Stir in pearl barley, vegetable broth, and dried thyme. After bringing to a simmer, cook until the barley is cooked, about 30 minutes.

4. Add pepper and salt to taste.

5. Serve hot, garnished with chopped fresh parsley.

Nutrition Information (per serving):

Calories: 220
Protein: 7g
Carbohydrates: 40g
Fat: 4g
Fiber: 9g
Sugar: 3g
Sodium: 600mg

Serving Size: 1 cup

These soups are nutritious, hearty, and full of flavor, making them perfect for individuals with Parkinson's disease. Dietary restrictions and personal preferences might be taken into consideration while making adjustments. Enjoy these comforting soups as part of a balanced meal or as a light meal on their own.

Chapter Three: Parkinson's Diet Salad

Quinoa Salad with Chickpeas and Vegetables:

Ingredients:

1 cup quinoa, rinsed
Two cups of veggie broth or water
Rinsed and drained chickpeas, one can (15 ounces)
1 cucumber, diced
1 bell pepper, diced
1 cup cherry tomatoes, halved
1/4 cup chopped fresh parsley
1/4 cup chopped fresh mint
2 tablespoons olive oil
2 tablespoons lemon juice
Salt and pepper to taste

Preparation Time: 15 minutes
Cooking Time: 15 minutes

Method of Preparation:

1. In a medium saucepan, combine quinoa and water or vegetable broth. Bring to a boil, then reduce heat to

low, cover, and simmer for 15 minutes, or until quinoa is cooked and water is absorbed. Take it off the fire and allow it to cool.

2. In a large bowl, combine cooked quinoa, chickpeas, diced cucumber, diced bell pepper, halved cherry tomatoes, chopped parsley, and chopped mint.

3. Combine lemon juice, olive oil, salt, and pepper in a small bowl and whisk together. After adding the dressing to the salad, toss to mix.

4. It can be served warm or cold.

Nutrition Information (per serving):

Calories: 280
Protein: 9g
Carbohydrates: 42g
Fat: 8g
Fiber: 7g
Sugar: 4g
Sodium: 320mg

Serving Size: 1 cup

<u>Spinach Salad with Strawberries and Almonds:</u>

Ingredients:

4 cups fresh spinach leaves
1 cup sliced strawberries
1/4 cup sliced almonds
2 tablespoons crumbled feta cheese (optional)
2 tablespoons balsamic vinegar
1 tablespoon olive oil
1 teaspoon honey
Salt and pepper to taste

Preparation Time: 10 minutes
Cooking Time: 0 minutes

Method of Preparation:

1. In a large bowl, combine fresh spinach leaves, sliced strawberries, sliced almonds, and crumbled feta cheese (if using).

2. In a small bowl, whisk together balsamic vinegar, olive oil, honey, salt, and pepper to make the dressing.

3. Drizzle the salad with the dressing and toss to evenly coat.

4. Serve immediately.

Nutrition Information (per serving):

Calories: 180
Protein: 5g
Carbohydrates: 14g
Fat: 12g
Fiber: 4g
Sugar: 7g
Sodium: 200mg

Serving Size: 2 cups

Mediterranean Chickpea Salad:

Ingredients:

Rinsed and drained chickpeas, one can (15 ounces)
1 cucumber, diced
1 bell pepper, diced
1 cup cherry tomatoes, halved
1/4 cup sliced Kalamata olives
1/4 cup of feta cheese, crumbled (optional)
2 tablespoons chopped fresh parsley
Two tablespoons of extra virgin olive oil.
1 tablespoon red wine vinegar
1 teaspoon dried oregano
Salt and pepper to taste

Preparation Time: 15 minutes
Cooking Time: 0 minutes

Method of Preparation:

1. In a large bowl, combine chickpeas, diced cucumber, diced bell pepper, halved cherry tomatoes, sliced Kalamata olives, crumbled feta cheese (if using), and chopped fresh parsley.

2. In a small bowl, whisk together extra virgin olive oil, red wine vinegar, dried oregano, salt, and pepper to make the dressing.

3. Drizzle the salad with the dressing and toss to evenly coat.

4. Serve right away or put in the fridge until you're ready to serve.

Nutrition Information (per serving):

Calories: 220
Protein: 8g
Carbohydrates: 22g
Fat: 12g
Fiber: 6g
Sugar: 4g
Sodium: 320mg
Serving Size: 1 cup

AsianInspired Quinoa Salad:

Ingredients:

1 cup quinoa, rinsed
Two cups of veggie broth or water
1 cup shredded cabbage
1 carrot, shredded
1 bell pepper, thinly sliced
1/4 cup chopped green onions
2 tablespoons chopped cilantro
2 tablespoons soy sauce (or tamari for a gluten-free option)
1 tablespoon rice vinegar
1 tablespoon sesame oil
1 teaspoon honey
1 teaspoon grated ginger
Sesame seeds for garnish (optional)

Preparation Time: 15 minutes
Cooking Time: 15 minutes

Method of Preparation:

1. In a medium saucepan, combine quinoa and water or vegetable broth. Bring to a boil, then reduce heat to low, cover, and simmer for 15 minutes, or until quinoa is

cooked and water is absorbed. Take it off the fire and allow it to cool.

2. In a large bowl, combine cooked quinoa, shredded cabbage, shredded carrot, thinly sliced bell pepper, chopped green onions, and chopped cilantro.

3. In a small bowl, whisk together soy sauce, rice vinegar, sesame oil, honey, and grated ginger to make the dressing.

4. Once the salad is evenly coated, drizzle with the dressing and toss.

5. If desired, sprinkle sesame seeds on top.

6. You can serve it cold or warm.

Nutrition Information (per serving):

Calories: 250
Protein: 7g
Carbohydrates: 36g
Fat: 8g
Fiber: 5g
Sugar: 5g
Sodium: 380mg

Serving Size: 1 cup

Of course! Here are two additional Parkinson's Friendly salad recipes:

Lemon Vinaigrette Kale and Quinoa Salad:

Ingredients:

1 cup quinoa, rinsed
Two cups of veggie broth or water
4 cups chopped kale leaves
1/2 cup cherry tomatoes, halved
1/4 cup sliced almonds
1/4 cup of feta cheese, crumbled (optional)
2 tablespoons olive oil
2 tablespoons lemon juice
1 teaspoon honey
1 teaspoon Dijon mustard
Salt and pepper to taste

Preparation Time: 15 minutes
Cooking Time: 15 minutes

Method of Preparation:

1. In a medium saucepan, combine quinoa and water or vegetable broth. Bring to a boil, then reduce heat to low, cover, and simmer for 15 minutes, or until quinoa is cooked and water is absorbed. Take it off the fire and allow it to cool.

2. In a large bowl, combine cooked quinoa, chopped kale leaves, halved cherry tomatoes, sliced almonds, and crumbled feta cheese (if using).

3. In a small bowl, whisk together olive oil, lemon juice, honey, Dijon mustard, salt, and pepper to make the vinaigrette.

4. Drizzle the vinaigrette over the salad and toss to coat evenly.

5. You can serve cold or room temperature.

Nutrition Information (per serving):

Calories: 280
Protein: 9g
Carbohydrates: 31g
Fat: 13g
Fiber: 5g
Sugar: 4g
Sodium: 230mg

Serving Size: 1 cup

<u>Tuna and White Bean Salad:</u>

Ingredients:

1 can (15 oz) white beans, drained and rinsed
1 can (5 oz) tuna, drained
1/4 cup diced red onion
1/4 cup chopped fresh parsley
1/4 cup chopped celery
1 tablespoon capers, drained
2 tablespoons olive oil
1 tablespoon lemon juice
Salt and pepper to taste

Preparation Time: 10 minutes
Cooking Time: 0 minutes

Method of Preparation:

1. In a large bowl, combine white beans, tuna, diced red onion, chopped fresh parsley, chopped celery, and capers.

2. In a small bowl, whisk together olive oil, lemon juice, salt, and pepper to make the dressing.

3. Drizzle the salad with the dressing and toss to evenly coat.

4. It can be served warm or cold.

Nutrition Information (per serving):

Calories: 270
Protein: 20g
Carbohydrates: 22g
Fat: 12g
Fiber: 6g
Sugar: 1g
Sodium: 350mg

Serving Size: 1 cup

These salads are nutritious, flavorful, and easy to prepare, making them perfect for individuals with Parkinson's disease. Dietary restrictions and personal preferences might be taken into consideration while making adjustments. Enjoy these delicious salads as a light meal or as a side dish with your favorite main course.

Chapter Four: Parkinson's Diet Main Dishes

Baked Salmon with Lemon Herb Crust:

Ingredients:

4 salmon filets
2 tablespoons olive oil
2 tablespoons fresh lemon juice
2 cloves garlic, minced
1 tablespoon chopped fresh parsley
1 teaspoon chopped fresh dill
Salt and pepper to taste
Lemon wedges for serving

Preparation Time: 10 minutes
Cooking Time: 15 minutes

Method of Preparation:

1. Preheat the oven to 400°F (200°C). Line a baking sheet with parchment paper.

2. In a small bowl, whisk together olive oil, lemon juice, minced garlic, chopped parsley, chopped dill, salt, and pepper to make the marinade.

3. Transfer the salmon fillets to the baking sheet that has been ready. Evenly brush the fish with the marinade.

4. Bake in the preheated oven for 12-15 minutes, or until the salmon is cooked through and flakes easily with a fork.

5. Serve hot, garnished with lemon wedges.

Nutrition Information (per serving):

Calories: 300
Protein: 25g
Carbohydrates: 2g
Fat: 20g
Fiber: 0g
Sugar: 0g
Sodium: 150mg

Serving Size: 1 salmon fillet

<u>Turkey and Vegetable StirFry:</u>

Ingredients:

1 pound thinly sliced turkey breast
Two tablespoons soy sauce (glutenfree option: tamari)
1 tablespoon hoisin sauce
1 tablespoon rice vinegar
1 tablespoon sesame oil
2 cloves garlic, minced
1 teaspoon grated ginger
1 bell pepper, thinly sliced
1 cup broccoli florets
1 carrot, thinly sliced
1/2 cup snap peas
Cooked brown rice for serving
Chopped green onions for garnish

Preparation Time: 15 minutes
Cooking Time: 15 minutes

Method of Preparation:

1. In a small bowl, whisk together soy sauce, hoisin sauce, rice vinegar, sesame oil, minced garlic, and grated ginger to make the sauce.

2. In a big wok or skillet over medium-high heat, heat up one tablespoon of oil. Add thinly sliced turkey breast and cook until browned and cooked through about 5-7 minutes. Take out of the skillet and place it aside.

3. In the same skillet, add a little more oil if needed. Add thinly sliced bell pepper, broccoli florets, sliced carrot, and snap peas. Stir Fry for 3-4 minutes, or until the vegetables are tender-crisp

4. Return the cooked turkey to the skillet and pour the sauce over the turkey and vegetables. Once coated evenly, stir and fully heat.

5. Serve the turkey and vegetable stir fry hot cooked brown rice. Garnish with chopped green onions.

Nutrition Information (per serving, without rice):

Calories: 250
Protein: 30g
Carbohydrates: 10g
Fat: 10g
Fiber: 3g
Sugar: 5g
Sodium: 600mg

Serving Size: 1 cup of stir fry

<u>Vegetable and Chickpea Curry:</u>

Ingredients:

1 tablespoon olive oil
1 onion, chopped
2 cloves garlic, minced
1 tablespoon curry powder
1 teaspoon ground cumin
1 teaspoon ground coriander
Rinsed and drained chickpeas, one can (15 ounces)
A single 14.5 oz can of chopped tomatoes
1 cup vegetable broth
2 cups chopped vegetables (such as bell peppers, carrots, and cauliflower)
Salt and pepper to taste
Cooked rice or quinoa for serving
Chopped fresh cilantro for garnish

Preparation Time: 15 minutes
Cooking Time: 25 minutes

Method of Preparation:

1. In a big skillet or pot, warm up the olive oil over medium heat. Add chopped onion and minced garlic, and cook until softened about 5 minutes.

2. Add curry powder, ground cumin, and ground coriander to the skillet, and cook for 1 minute, stirring constantly.

3. Stir in drained chickpeas, diced tomatoes (with their juices), vegetable broth, and chopped vegetables. Season with salt and pepper to taste.

4. Bring the mixture to a simmer, then reduce heat to low. Cover and cook for 15-20 minutes, or until the vegetables are tender.

5. Serve the vegetable and chickpea curry hot overcooked rice or quinoa. Garnish with chopped fresh cilantro.

Nutrition Information (per serving, without rice/quinoa):

Calories: 220
Protein: 8g
Carbohydrates: 32g
Fat: 7g
Fiber: 8g
Sugar: 6g
Sodium: 500mg

Serving Size: 1 cup of curry

Baked Chicken with Roasted Vegetables:

Ingredients:

4 boneless, skinless chicken breasts
2 tablespoons olive oil
1 teaspoon dried Italian seasoning
1/2 teaspoon garlic powder
1/2 teaspoon onion powder
Salt and pepper to taste
2 cups chopped vegetables (such as bell peppers, zucchini, and red onion)

Preparation Time: 10 minutes
Cooking Time: 25 minutes

Method of Preparation:

1. Preheat the oven to 400°F (200°C). Line a baking sheet with parchment paper.

2. Transfer the chicken breasts to the baking sheet that has been ready. Drizzle with olive oil and sprinkle with dried Italian seasoning, garlic powder, onion powder, salt, and pepper.

3. Arrange chopped vegetables around the chicken on the baking sheet. Sprinkle it with salt and pepper and drizzle with olive oil.

4. Bake in the preheated oven for 20-25 minutes, or until the chicken is cooked through and the vegetables are tender.

5. Serve the baked chicken with roasted vegetables hot, as is, or with a side salad.

Nutrition Information (per serving):

Calories: 250
Protein: 30g
Carbohydrates: 10g
Fat: 10g
Fiber: 3g
Sugar: 5g
Sodium: 300mg

Serving Size: 1 chicken breast with vegetables

<u>Vegetable StirFried Noodles:</u>

Ingredients:

Eight ounces of brown rice or whole-wheat pasta
2 tablespoons sesame oil
1 onion, thinly sliced
2 cloves garlic, minced
1 bell pepper, thinly sliced
1 carrot, julienned
2 cups broccoli florets
1 cup snap peas
1/4 cup low-sodium soy sauce (or tamari for a gluten-free option)
2 tablespoons rice vinegar
1 tablespoon honey
1 teaspoon grated ginger
Sesame seeds for garnish (optional)
Preparation Time: 15 minutes
Cooking Time: 15 minutes

Method of Preparation:

1. Cook noodles according to package instructions. Drain and set aside.

2. In a large skillet or wok, heat sesame oil over medium-high heat. Add thinly sliced onion and minced garlic, and cook until fragrant, about 1 minute.

3. Fill the skillet with snap peas, broccoli florets, julienned carrot, and thinly sliced bell pepper. When the vegetables are crisp-tender, stir-fry them for five to seven minutes.

4. Combine the soy sauce, rice vinegar, honey, and grated ginger to make the sauce.

5. Add cooked noodles to the skillet, pour the sauce over the noodles and vegetables, and toss to combine.

6. Cook for an additional 2-3 minutes, or until heated through.

7. Serve the vegetable stir-fried noodles hot, garnished with sesame seeds if desired.

Nutrition Information (per serving):
Calories: 350

Protein: 10g
Carbohydrates: 60g
Fat: 8g
Fiber: 10g
Sugar: 10g
Sodium: 600mg

Serving Size: 1 cup of noodles with vegetables

Mediterranean Grilled Chicken Skewers:

Ingredients:

1 lb boneless, skinless chicken breasts, cut into cubes
1 tablespoon olive oil
2 cloves garlic, minced
1 teaspoon dried oregano
1 teaspoon dried thyme
1 teaspoon dried rosemary
Juice of 1 lemon
Salt and pepper to taste
Cherry tomatoes
Red onion, cut into chunks
Bell peppers, cut into chunks

Preparation Time: 20 minutes
Cooking Time: 10 minutes

Method of Preparation:

1. In a bowl, combine olive oil, minced garlic, dried oregano, dried thyme, dried rosemary, lemon juice, salt, and pepper to make the marinade.

2. Add cubed chicken breast to the marinade, toss to coat evenly, cover, and refrigerate for at least 30 minutes.

3. Preheat the grill to medium-high heat. Thread marinated chicken cubes onto skewers, alternating with cherry tomatoes, chunks of red onion, and chunks of bell peppers.

4. Grill skewers for 4-5 minutes on each side, or until the chicken is cooked through and has grill marks.

5. Serve the Mediterranean grilled chicken skewers hot with a side of your favorite salad or whole grain.

Nutrition Information (per serving):

Calories: 250
Protein: 30g
Carbohydrates: 10g
Fat: 10g
Fiber: 3g
Sugar: 5g
Sodium: 300mg

Serving Size: 2 skewers

These main dishes are flavorful, balanced, and easy to prepare, making them ideal for individuals with Parkinson's disease. Dietary restrictions and personal preferences might be taken into consideration while making adjustments. Savor these mouthwatering dishes as a part of a healthy diet.

Chapter Five: Parkinson's Diet Side Dishes

Roasted Garlic Mashed Cauliflower:

Ingredients:

1 head cauliflower, chopped into florets
3 cloves garlic, minced
2 tablespoons olive oil
Salt and pepper to taste
Chopped fresh chives for garnish

Preparation Time: 10 minutes
Cooking Time: 25 minutes

Method of Preparation:

1. Preheat the oven to 400°F (200°C). Line a baking sheet with parchment paper.

2. In a large bowl, toss cauliflower florets and minced garlic with olive oil until evenly coated. Season with salt and pepper.

3. Spread the cauliflower mixture in a single layer on the prepared baking sheet.

4. Roast in the preheated oven for 20-25 minutes, or until the cauliflower is tender and lightly browned, stirring halfway through.

5. Transfer the roasted cauliflower and garlic to a food processor. Pulse until smooth and creamy.

6. Serve the roasted garlic mashed cauliflower hot, garnished with chopped fresh chives.

Nutrition Information (per serving):

Calories: 100
Protein: 3g
Carbohydrates: 8g
Fat: 7g
Fiber: 4g
Sugar: 3g
Sodium: 40mg

Serving Size: 1/2 cup

<u>Quinoa and Vegetable Pilaf:</u>

Ingredients:

1 cup quinoa, rinsed
Two cups of veggie broth or water
1 tablespoon olive oil
1 onion, chopped
2 cloves garlic, minced
1 bell pepper, diced
1 carrot, diced
1 cup frozen peas
1/4 cup chopped fresh parsley
Salt and pepper to taste

Preparation Time: 10 minutes
Cooking Time: 20 minutes

Method of Preparation:

1. In a medium saucepan, combine quinoa and water or vegetable broth. Once you have brought the quinoa to a boil, lower the heat to a simmer, cover, and let it cook for 15 to 20 minutes, or until the water has been absorbed. Take it off the stove and give it a little time to cool.

2. In a large skillet, heat olive oil over medium heat. Add chopped onion and minced garlic, and cook until softened about 5 minutes.

3. Add diced bell pepper, diced carrot, and frozen peas to the skillet. Cook for another 5 minutes, or until vegetables are tender.

4. Stir cooked quinoa into the skillet with the vegetables. Cook for a further two to three minutes, stirring now and then.

5. Season with salt and pepper to taste, and stir in chopped fresh parsley.

6. Serve the quinoa and vegetable pilaf hot as a side dish or as a base for protein.

Nutrition Information (per serving):

Calories: 180
Protein: 5g
Carbohydrates: 30g
Fat: 5g
Fiber: 6g
Sugar: 4g
Sodium: 50mg

Serving Size: 1/2 cup

Garlic Herb Roasted Potatoes:

Ingredients:

1 lb baby potatoes, halved
2 tablespoons olive oil
3 cloves garlic, minced
1 teaspoon dried thyme
1 teaspoon dried rosemary
Salt and pepper to taste
Chopped fresh parsley for garnish

Preparation Time: 10 minutes
Cooking Time: 30 minutes

Method of Preparation:

1. Preheat the oven to 400°F (200°C). Line a baking sheet with parchment paper.

2. In a large bowl, toss halved baby potatoes with olive oil, minced garlic, dried thyme, dried rosemary, salt, and pepper until evenly coated.

3. Spread the seasoned potatoes in a single layer on the prepared baking sheet.

4. Roast in the preheated oven for 25-30 minutes, or until the potatoes are golden brown and tender, stirring halfway through.

5. Transfer the roasted potatoes to a serving dish, garnish with chopped fresh parsley, and serve hot.

Nutrition Information (per serving):

Calories: 150
Protein: 2g
Carbohydrates: 20g
Fat: 7g
Fiber: 2g
Sugar: 1g
Sodium: 10mg

Serving Size: 1/2 cup

Sauteed Garlic Green Beans:

Ingredients:

1 lb green beans, trimmed
2 tablespoons olive oil
3 cloves garlic, minced
Salt and pepper to taste
Lemon wedges for serving

Preparation Time: 10 minutes
Cooking Time: 10 minutes

Method of Preparation:

1. Heat up some salted water in a pot. Add trimmed green beans and blanch for 2-3 minutes, or until bright green and crisp-tender. Drain and set aside.

2. In a large skillet, heat olive oil over medium heat. Add the minced garlic and simmer for one minute or until fragrant.

3. Add blanched green beans to the skillet and sauté for 57 minutes, or until tender but still crisp.

4. Add pepper and salt to taste.

5. Serve the sautéed garlic green beans hot, with lemon wedges on the side for squeezing.

Nutrition Information (per serving):

Calories: 80
Protein: 2g
Carbohydrates: 7g
Fat: 6g
Fiber: 3g
Sugar: 2g
Sodium: 5mg

Serving Size: 1/2 cup

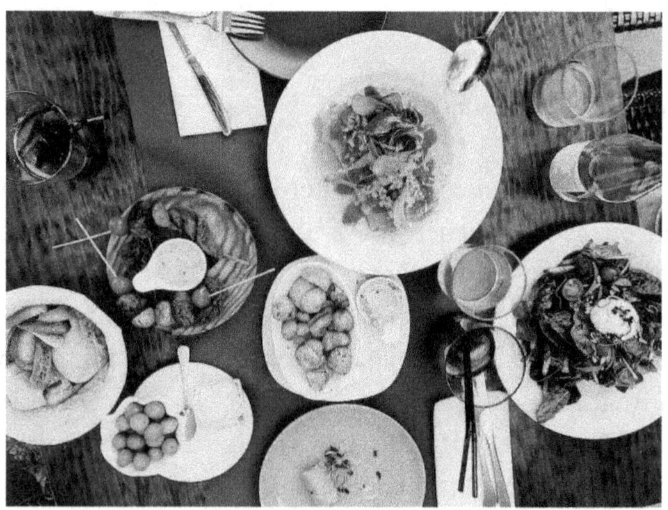

Quinoa Stuffed Bell Peppers:

Ingredients:

4 bell peppers, any color
1 cup quinoa, rinsed
2 cups vegetable broth
1 tablespoon olive oil
1 onion, diced
2 cloves garlic, minced
1 cup diced tomatoes
1 cup cooked black beans
1 teaspoon ground cumin
1 teaspoon smoked paprika
Salt and pepper to taste
Chopped fresh cilantro for garnish

Preparation Time: 15 minutes
Cooking Time: 40 minutes

Method of Preparation:

1. Preheat the oven to 375°F (190°C). Slice the tops off the bell peppers and remove the seeds and membranes. Place the bell peppers in a baking dish.

2. Add the vegetable broth and quinoa to a medium-sized saucepan. Bring to a boil, then reduce heat

to low, cover, and simmer for 15-20 minutes, or until quinoa is cooked and liquid is absorbed. Remove from heat and set aside.

3. Add the olive oil to a skillet and heat it to medium. Add diced onion and minced garlic, and cook until softened about 5 minutes.

4. Stir in diced tomatoes, cooked black beans, ground cumin, smoked paprika, cooked quinoa, salt, and pepper. Add another 5 minutes of cooking and stir from time to time.

5. Spoon the quinoa mixture into the prepared bell peppers.

6. Bake in the preheated oven for 20-25 minutes, or until the bell peppers are tender.

7. Garnish with chopped fresh cilantro before serving.

Nutrition Information (per serving, based on 1 stuffed bell pepper):

Calories: 250
Protein: 9g
Carbohydrates: 45g
Fat: 5g
Fiber: 10g
Sugar: 7g
Sodium: 480mg
Serving Quantity: 1 whole bell pepper

Sautéed Spinach with Garlic and Lemon:

Ingredients:

1 lb fresh spinach leaves, washed and trimmed
2 tablespoons olive oil
3 cloves garlic, minced
Juice of 1 lemon
Salt and pepper to taste

Preparation Time: 5 minutes
Cooking Time: 5 minutes

Method of Preparation:

1. Heat olive oil in a large skillet over medium heat. Add the minced garlic and simmer for one minute or until fragrant.

2. Add fresh spinach leaves to the skillet, a handful at a time, and toss until wilted. Continue adding spinach until it's all wilted.

3. Squeeze lemon juice over the spinach and season with salt and pepper to taste. Toss to combine.

4. Cook for another 2-3 minutes, or until the spinach is heated through.

5. Serve the sautéed spinach hot as a nutritious side dish.

Nutrition Information (per serving):

Calories: 80
Protein: 5g
Carbohydrates: 4g
Fat: 6g
Fiber: 3g
Sugar: 0g
Sodium: 90mg

Serving Size: 1 cup

These side dishes are nutritious, flavorful, and easy to prepare, making them perfect additions to any meal for individuals with Parkinson's disease. Dietary restrictions and personal preferences might be taken into consideration while making adjustments. Enjoy these delicious sides as part of a balanced diet.

Chapter Six: Parkinson's Diet Dessert

Banana Oat Cookies:

Ingredients:

2 ripe bananas, mashed
1 cup rolled oats
1/4 cup unsweetened applesauce
1/4 cup chopped nuts (such as walnuts or almonds)
1/4 cup raisins or dried cranberries
1 teaspoon ground cinnamon
1/2 teaspoon vanilla extract

Preparation Time: 10 minutes
Cooking Time: 15 minutes

Method of Preparation:

1. Preheat the oven to 350°F (175°C). Line a baking sheet with parchment paper.
2. In a large bowl, combine mashed bananas, rolled oats, unsweetened applesauce, chopped nuts, raisins or dried cranberries, ground cinnamon, and vanilla extract. Mix well to combine.

3. Drop spoonfuls of the cookie dough onto the prepared baking sheet, spacing them apart.

4. Flatten each cookie slightly with the back of a spoon.

5. Bake in the preheated oven for 15-18 minutes, or until the cookies are golden brown and set.

6. After a few minutes of cooling on the baking sheet, move the cookies to a wire rack to finish cooling.

Nutrition Information (per serving, based on 1 cookie):

Calories: 70
Protein: 1g
Carbohydrates: 12g
Fat: 2g
Fiber: 2g
Sugar: 4g
Sodium: 0mg

Serving Size: 1 cookie

<u>Berry Yogurt Parfait:</u>

Ingredients:

1 cup plain Greek yogurt
1/2 cup mixed berries (such as strawberries, blueberries, and raspberries)
1 tablespoon honey
1/4 cup granola
Fresh mint leaves for garnish (optional)

Preparation Time: 5 minutes
Cooking Time: 0 minutes
Method of Preparation:

1. In a glass or serving dish, layer plain Greek yogurt, mixed berries, and granola.
2. Drizzle honey over the top of the parfait.
Add some fresh mint leaves as a garnish if preferred.
4. Serve the berry yogurt parfait immediately as a delicious and refreshing dessert.

Nutrition Information (per serving):

Calories: 200
Protein: 15g
Carbohydrates: 30g

Fat: 4g
Fiber: 4g
Sugar: 16g
Sodium: 60mg

Serving Size: 1 parfait

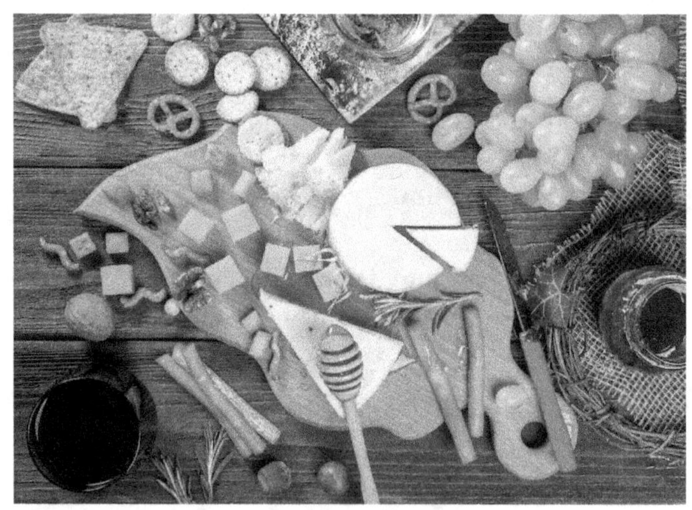

Baked Apples with Cinnamon and Walnuts:

Ingredients:

4 apples, cored
1/4 cup chopped walnuts
Two teaspoons of maple syrup or honey
1 teaspoon ground cinnamon
1/4 teaspoon ground nutmeg
1/4 cup apple juice or water

Preparation Time: 10 minutes
Cooking Time: 30 minutes

Method of Preparation:

1. Preheat the oven to 375°F (190°C).
2. In a small bowl, combine chopped walnuts, honey or maple syrup, ground cinnamon, and ground nutmeg.
3. Place cored apples in a baking dish. Fill each apple cavity with the walnut mixture.
4. Pour water or apple juice into the bottom of the baking dish.
5. Cover the baking dish with foil and bake in the preheated oven for 20-25 minutes.
6. Take off the foil and continue baking the apples for a further five to ten minutes, or until they are soft.

7. Serve the baked apples hot, optionally with a dollop of Greek yogurt or a sprinkle of additional cinnamon on top.

Nutrition Information (per serving):

Calories: 150
Protein: 2g
Carbohydrates: 30g
Fat: 4g
Fiber: 5g
Sugar: 22g
Sodium: 0mg

Serving Size: 1 baked apple

<u>Chocolate Avocado Mousse:</u>

Ingredients:

Two mature avocados, seeded and deseeded
1/4 cup cocoa powder
1/4 cup maple syrup or honey
1 teaspoon vanilla extract
Pinch of salt
Fresh berries for garnish (optional)

Preparation Time: 10 minutes
Cooking Time: 0 minutes

Method of Preparation:

1. In a food processor or blender, combine ripe avocados, cocoa powder, honey or maple syrup, vanilla extract, and a pinch of salt.

2. Process until creamy and smooth, scraping down the sides as necessary.

3. Taste and adjust sweetness if needed by adding more honey or maple syrup.

4. Transfer the chocolate avocado mousse to serving dishes.

5. Before serving, let the food cool for at least half an hour in the refrigerator.

6. Garnish with fresh berries before serving if desired.

Nutrition Information (per serving):

Calories: 200
Protein: 3g
Carbohydrates: 20g
Fat: 15g
Fiber: 7g
Sugar: 12g
Sodium: 5mg

Serving Measurement: 1/2 cup mousse

Frozen Banana Bites:

Ingredients:

2 ripe bananas, peeled and sliced into rounds
1/4 cup peanut butter or almond butter
1/4 cup dark chocolate chips
1 tablespoon coconut oil
Chopped nuts or shredded coconut for garnish (optional)

Preparation Time: 15 minutes
Cooking Time: 0 minutes

Method of Preparation:

1. Line a baking sheet with parchment paper.

2. Spread a small amount of peanut butter or almond butter on half of the banana slices, then sandwich them with the other half of the slices to form banana bites.

3. Place the banana bites on the prepared baking sheet and freeze for at least 30 minutes.

4. In a microwave-safe bowl, combine dark chocolate chips and coconut oil. When the chocolate is smooth and melted, microwave it for 30-second bursts, stirring every 30 seconds.

5. Remove the frozen banana bites from the freezer and dip each one halfway into the melted chocolate, then place them back on the baking sheet.

6. Sprinkle chopped nuts or shredded coconut on top of the chocolate-dipped banana bites if desired.

7. Return the banana bites to the freezer and freeze until the chocolate is set for about 1 hour.

8. Serve the frozen banana bites cold as a delicious and refreshing treat.

Nutrition Information (per serving, based on 4 banana bites):

Calories: 150
Protein: 3g
Carbohydrates: 20g
Fat: 8g
Fiber: 3g
Sugar: 12g
Sodium: 20mg

Serving Size: 4 banana bites

<u>Mixed Berry Sorbet:</u>

Ingredients:

2 cups mixed berries (such as strawberries, blueberries, and raspberries), frozen
One tablespoon of maple syrup or honey, optional depending on how sweet the berries are.
1 tablespoon lemon juice
Fresh mint leaves for garnish (optional)

Preparation Time: 5 minutes
Cooking Time: 0 minutes

Method of Preparation:

1. In a blender or food processor, combine frozen mixed berries, honey or maple syrup (if using), and lemon juice.
2. Process until creamy and smooth, scraping down the sides as necessary.
3. Taste and adjust sweetness if needed by adding more honey or maple syrup.
4. Transfer the mixed berry mixture to a shallow dish and spread it out evenly.
5. Freeze for at least 2 hours, or until firm.

6. Using a fork, scrape the frozen mixture to create a sorbet-like texture.

7. Serve the mixed berry sorbet in bowls, garnished with fresh mint leaves if desired.

Nutrition Information (per serving, based on 1/2 cup):

Calories: 60
Protein: 1g
Carbohydrates: 15g
Fat: 0g
Fiber: 3g
Sugar: 10g
Sodium: 0mg

Serving Size: 1/2 cup

These dessert options are refreshing, satisfying, and easy to prepare, making them perfect treats for individuals with Parkinson's disease. Dietary restrictions and personal preferences might be taken into consideration while making adjustments. Enjoy these delightful desserts as a guilt-free indulgence!

Tips for eating out safely

Eating out can be enjoyable, but it's essential for individuals with Parkinson's disease to ensure their meals are safe and suitable for their needs. Here are some tips for eating out safely:

1. Plan Ahead: Research restaurants in advance to find ones that offer Parkinson 's-friendly options or accommodations such as quieter environments, flexible seating arrangements, or menus with clear labeling of ingredients.

2. Communicate: Inform the restaurant staff about any dietary restrictions or special needs due to Parkinson's disease. They can often accommodate requests for modifications to dishes, such as cooking methods or ingredient substitutions.

3. Choose Wisely: Look for dishes that are easy to eat, such as grilled or baked options, steamed vegetables, soups, or salads. Avoid foods that are difficult to handle or chew, overly spicy, or high in sodium.

4. Ask Questions: Don't hesitate to ask about how dishes are prepared, including cooking methods, ingredients, and portion sizes. It's essential to be aware of any potential triggers or allergens.

5. Portion Control: Consider ordering smaller portions or sharing dishes with dining companions to avoid overeating and minimize the risk of digestive issues or discomfort.

6. Stay Hydrated: Drink water or other nonalcoholic beverages throughout the meal to stay hydrated and aid digestion. Limit alcohol consumption, as it can interact with medications and exacerbate Parkinson's symptoms.

7. Be Mindful of Medications: If you take medication that requires specific timing with meals, plan your dining experience accordingly to ensure you can take your medication as prescribed.

8. Take Your Time: Eat slowly and pace yourself to avoid swallowing difficulties or choking hazards associated with Parkinson's disease. Chew thoroughly and take breaks between bites if needed.

9. Be Prepared: Consider bringing utensils or adaptive devices if you have difficulty with fine motor skills or gripping utensils. Portable utensil sets or specialized utensils designed for individuals with Parkinson's can be helpful.

10. Listen to Your Body: Pay attention to how your body responds to different foods and dining experiences. If you experience any discomfort or symptoms, take appropriate action and seek assistance if necessary.

By following these tips and being proactive in your dining choices, you can enjoy eating out safely and comfortably while managing Parkinson's disease effectively.

Wait a moment! Before you leave...

I trust this cookbook has offered you inspiration, comfort, and value. Each recipe was crafted with love, attention to detail, and a deep understanding of utilizing Parkinson's recipes for crafting wholesome meals.

Your reviews, experiences, and insights are invaluable to me. Each evaluation propels my growth, helping me tailor my work to better suit your needs. It's a dialogue, a connection that extends beyond the written word.
With sincere gratitude and anticipation

Conclusion

As the journey through the pages of this book draws to a close, it is with a sense of profound gratitude and hope that I bid farewell to you, dear reader. Throughout these chapters, we have delved into the intricate nuances of Parkinson's disease, exploring its multifaceted impact on both body and mind. We have navigated through the complexities of symptom management, uncovering the power of nutrition as a pivotal tool in enhancing quality of life and mitigating the challenges posed by this condition.

But beyond the realm of mere dietary guidelines and culinary explorations, we have unearthed a deeper truth: the resilience of the human spirit in the face of adversity. In the stories shared and the voices heard, we have witnessed the unwavering courage and determination of individuals living with Parkinson's, as well as their caregivers and loved ones, who stand steadfast in their support.

As the final chapter closes, let us carry forth the wisdom gleaned from these pages as a testament to the indomitable strength that resides within each of us. May we continue to journey forward with compassion, understanding, and a steadfast commitment to fostering a world where those affected by Parkinson's disease are met with unwavering support and boundless opportunities for healing and growth.

In closing, I extend my heartfelt gratitude to all who have embarked on this literary voyage with me. May the insights gained serve as guiding beacons of light, illuminating the path toward a brighter, more compassionate future for all. With deepest sincerity and warmest wishes, I bid you adieu until we meet again on the next chapter of life's extraordinary journey.

www.ingramcontent.com/pod-product-compliance
Lightning Source LLC
Chambersburg PA
CBHW050833260726

48660CB00006B/2208